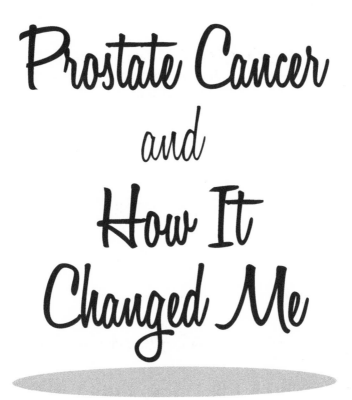

Prostate Cancer
and
How It
Changed Me

William J. Voller, Jr.

PAGE PUBLISHING
Conneaut Lake, PA

First originally published by Page Publishing 2022

ISBN 978-1-6624-8047-8 (pbk)
ISBN 978-1-6624-8048-5 (digital)

Printed in the United States of America

To my beautiful wife, Cory. She was and is
my rock and support. I love her so.

So you have prostate cancer...

Contents

Introduction

I am writing this story to tell how prostate cancer impacted my life and the lives of the loved ones surrounding me. There are many books out about how breast cancer affects women. In fact, I was watching television while I was running on a treadmill earlier this month, and there was another women author being interviewed on her book about breast cancer. I think it is terrific that breast cancer has the support that it has, but I think it is about time that prostate cancer, the number one cancer killer of males, has some equal information sharing.

When I was diagnosed with prostate cancer, there was no place to turn for actual information that was experienced-based. There was a great deal of information on the internet, but no one that I could turn to ask questions. I could not find any books on the subject that were not written by a doctor and were very technical in nature.

Please do not use this book as the bible on prostate cancer. It is just an outpouring of my experiences. It is *not* to be used as a guide or the correct way to go. The options I selected worked for my situation and me. They may not work for you. I really just wanted to get my experience down on paper so others could read it and maybe be more comfortable with the process. Prostate cancer is a bad reality. I hope those that read this book have a better feel for what lies ahead for them so that, the more information you have, the better decisions can be made.

In November of 2014, my father, William John Voller, died of complications due to prostate cancer. He was ninety-seven years old. When he died, his PSA score was over 200!

I have changed the names of the doctors I worked with during this process as well as the names of the hospitals they worked for.

Part 1

(February, March, April 2003)

Chapter 1

Prostate Cancer
Results of My First PSA Test

I can remember the telephone call very clearly. It was early in the morning, Monday, February 10, 2003. I was at work, sitting in my office. The phone rang, and I looked at the telephone number. I recognized the number as my doctor, Dr. John Jones, an Internist with a large hospital in Chicago. Due to my level at my company, a utility serving Chicagoland, I was set up with this intern organization for regularly scheduled physicals. I started seeing various interns in that group in June of 1996. I liked Dr. Jones. He was about my age, and he had a nice, calm manner. I saw him for most of my annual physicals.

I had turned fifty in late 2002. I was aware that I had been somewhat overweight, and I didn't like it. In fact, I was fat. As a result, my cholesterol was high, and my blood pressure was bad. I made the commitment in 2002 to get in shape. I told my beautiful wife, Cory, that by the end of 2002, she would "have the man back that she married in 1978."

I started exercising in March of 2002, and by the end of 2002, I had logged over seven hundred miles of running. I liked to run and had some success in the past losing weight via running. I tried to put in about three miles per day, sometimes swimming a quarter mile a day also.

I had discovered a fitness test devised by a well-known exercise specialist. This aerobic fitness test involved running a moderate distance as fast as you could. The specialist had identified several fitness categories: the best being *excellent*. He had correlated running times in a number of age groups, including fifty and above. My goal was to be in the *excellent* category in the fifty-plus age group by the time I turned fifty on December 10.

As the days went by and it got closer to December 10, I was running faster and faster. On November 16, 2002, I ran a distance in a time that was in the excellent category for my age—forty years old and above. On the day of my fiftieth birthday, December 10, 2002, I ran the same distance, now in the *excellent* category for the fifty-plus age group.

As I exercised and reached my goal, the weight dropped off. I had scheduled my annual physical for Thursday, February 6, 2003. I had lost over twenty-five pounds and was proud of my weight loss. I expected good results from the tests. However, there was a new test that Dr. Jones administered to me that day. He called it the PSA test, and he said it was regularly done for men fifty years old and older.

I had gotten cocky. I was in good shape and expected good news. Then right when I least expected it, the bottom fell out.

Back to the telephone call. I knew it couldn't be good. Any time a doctor calls you, it usually is bad news. As expected, Dr. Jones complimented me on my weight loss and recognized my excellent blood pressure and cholesterol results. He said there was a little problem with the results of the PSA test. My PSA score was high—8.0. However, he stated that there were many "false positives" (I never heard that term before) with the PSA, and he recommended that I come in again and take another PSA test. I asked what the PSA test was, and he stated that it was used to identify prostate cancer.

That was all I needed to hear, and really it was all I did hear. My mind went blank, and there was a buzzing in my ears. I kept on asking Dr. Jones, "What is prostate cancer?"

They say that when you are first diagnosed as having cancer, you believe you are going to die soon. That was exactly what I did. My mind rushed with how much time I had left, how I was going to die, what my family was going to do.

I couldn't work for the rest of the day. I needed to tell my family—my wife and my sons. I was a mess. I worried about cancer. I dreamed about having cancer—about dying early. I did tons of research on cancer and specifically prostate cancer.

At the same time, my dad called to tell me that my mom had been diagnosed with lung cancer. My mother had smoked early in life up until I was born. She had smoked while carrying me but gave up soon after my birth. However, she smoked nonfilter cigarettes—the worst kind.

I scheduled the follow-up test for later that week, Thursday, February 13, 2003.

Chapter 2

Follow-up Additional PSA Tests

I met with Dr. Jones and his team that week to take another PSA Test. The test is literally a "no-brainer." It is completed with a simple blood test. I had hoped that the first test result was a "false positive," as Dr. Jones had suggested. However, this test result not only confirmed the original high PSA count, but it had got higher. This result was an 8.5 PSA score.

What exactly does this PSA mean? *Prostate-specific antigen* or *PSA* is a protein produced by cells of the prostate gland. The PSA test measures the level of PSA in a man's blood. Test results are reported as nanograms of PSA per milliliter (ng/mL) of blood. The blood level of PSA is often elevated in men with prostate cancer. This test is usually administered to men beginning at the age of fifty. PSA scores of 4.0 ng/mL and lower are considered normal. A PSA score above 4.0 ng/mL may result in a doctor recommending a prostate biopsy. PSA scores between 4.0 and 10.0 ng/mL are considered mildly elevated and may suggest further review.

My two scores of 8.0 and 8.5 were both in the mildly elevated level. Dr. Jones recommended that I set up a visit with one of the best urologists in the country, Dr. Frank M. Smith, at the department of urology at one of the largest hospitals in Chicago. Dr. Jones knew Dr. Smith and spoke to him about me. An introductory appointment was set up for February 27, 2003, about two weeks after my second PSA test with Dr. Jones.

I was pretty nervous during that time and spent much of my free time reading as much as I could online on the prostate and prostate cancer. I tried to keep focused on my job and my family, but the prostate issue crept up, especially when there were no other issues for me to focus on.

I couldn't wait to meet Dr. Smith and discuss the next steps.

February 27, 2003, came soon enough. Dr. Smith was an older gentleman—tall and slender with a confidence of a doctor who knew his craft. I didn't exactly like him, but I respected his knowledge and experience. He didn't quite have Dr. Jones's patient rapport, but it was evident that he knew his stuff.

First things first, a digital rectal exam (gotta love 'em) and another PSA blood test. Dr. Smith suggested that we wait until he has the results of that test before we talk and make plans for the next steps.

Well, this PSA test didn't change things—the result was a score of 8.4, very consistent with the other two PSA tests that I had.

Dr. Smith called me after March 10, 2003, and we talked about options and suggestions for what to do next. He suggested that I undergo a prostate biopsy, which would confirm cancer in the prostate. He stated that there could be other reasons for high PSA counts. Very thick skin on the outside of the prostate has resulted in high PSA counts also. I agreed, and the biopsy was scheduled one month later, on March 26, 2003.

Chapter 3

The Biopsy Confirming Prostate Cancer Gleason Scores

If you think I was nervous before this, I was a confirmed basket case during the time before the biopsy. I had never had a biopsy before, and I was very concerned and anxious. My wife said I was an asshole to live with during this time.

The day of the biopsy came, and my wife, Cory, and I drove downtown together. I soon found out that I had a reason to be nervous. My name was called by the receptionist soon after I arrived, and I stepped into Dr. Smith's office, or should I say, "Torture chamber." The scene was right out of a Frankenstein movie. I actually laughed. On a shelf in his office, someone had spread out the tools that Dr. Smith could use or was going to use for this procedure. Wow, there were a lot of them! And these instruments were long, cold and looked evil.

Dr. Smith and his attending nurse explained what the biopsy entailed. First, the prostate had to be numbed. The prostate is a small gland about the size of a walnut sitting below a man's bladder. Dr. Smith was going to give me a shot in the prostate to numb it so he could take core samples of the prostate without me going through the roof. The tool that he used to give me that shot was several inches long and needed to be administered through my rectum. There was another tool to expand the rectum while the shot was going in. The most painful process was this first shot. My prostate had sat in my body undisturbed for over fifty years, and now someone was going to shoot it up with Novocain so it could be numb to the removal of the core plugs.

The shot hurt a lot!

Then Dr. Smith and his nurse explained exactly how they were going to harvest the core samples and what I should expect. They were going to use a tool that was essentially a tiny shovel if you will. The goal, Dr. Smith explained, was to obtain about eight cores on either side of my prostate.

The tool that Dr. Smith was using is actually called a *biopsy gun* and sounded very much like the cap gun we used when we were kids each time he pulled the trigger. With each trigger pull, the gun made a loud bang, and the tool pushed into my prostate and pulled out a core. Dr. Smith pulled out eight cores of tissue from the right side of my prostate, measuring 6.5 cm in aggregate length and 0.1 cm in diameter. He pulled out nine cores from the left side of my prostate, measuring 6.8 cm in aggregate length and 0.1 cm in diameter. The entire process took about half an hour in total time. Every time Dr. Smith took out a core, he said that it looked pretty good. I will say that I felt a slight punch in the rectum each time he pulled out a core plug, and my stomach was nauseated by the time the process was complete.

It didn't end there. After he was complete, he gave me a pad to place inside my underwear. He said that I would be bleeding for a while. He told me that he would contact me immediately after the analysis was complete to determine the state of my prostate—either cancerous or benign.

I walked out of the waiting room to my wife. Cory said I was white as a ghost. I felt miserable and went right to bed after getting home.

The waiting game began again. Needless to say, I was concerned. The results were completed at 6:38 p.m. on March 28, 2003. Dr. Smith reached out to me the next morning on March 29, 2003, with a summary of the findings.

The results of the needle core biopsy on the right side of my prostate were prostatic parenchyma with adenocarcinoma, Gleason scores 3+4, involving about 20 percent of the total submitted core

and showing focal perineural lesion in the small nerve. The results of
the needle core biopsy on the left side of my prostate were similar—
prostatic parenchyma with adenocarcinoma, Gleason scores 3+3,
involving approximately 20 percent of the total submitted prostate
cores.

It was finally confirmed, I had prostate cancer. Believe it or not,
I was somewhat relieved. I finally had an answer and now knew what
direction I had to go.

But still, now that I knew I had cancer, questions raced thru my
brain: how did I get it, am I contagious, why me?

Let's talk a little bit about the technical terms above. The most
important is the Gleason score.

The Gleason score correlates with the tumor's behavior. A low
score (2, 3, or 4) indicates a low-grade tumor. A midrange score (5,
6, or 7) indicates a moderate-grade tumor. A high score (8, 9, or
10) indicates a very aggressive tumor likely to come back even if
removed. My scores were 6 (3 + 3) and 7 (3 + 4) and are the most
frequent scores that doctors see. They usually indicate an average or
intermediate grade situation.

The Gleason scale is the most common grading scale for the
comparison of tumors. Cancer cells are assigned a certain point value,
if you will, based upon some well-accepted standards. The actual
criteria are twofold: one—how the cancer cells look and two—how
they are arranged together. Each component is given a score from 1
to 5. The two numbers are added together to determine the Gleason
sum. As I stated above, my scores were 6 and 7.

High-grade cancers are the deadly ones. They show up on the
Gleason scale as scores equaling 8, 9, and 10. They are hard to treat
and quick to come back. Some do not respond to hormone therapy at all. They tend to be large, rapid-growing, very aggressive, and
quick to grow into surrounding tissues.

Intermediate-grade Gleason scores are in the 5, 6, or 7 range on
the Gleason scale. They can contain either low-grade or high-grade
scores, depending on how much tumor volume is present and how
high the PSA is. A Gleason score of 7 is more aggressive than a score
of 6 but less aggressive than high-grade cancers. To make things even

more confusing a Gleason score of 7 composed of 3 + 4 is better than a Gleason score of 7 composed of 4 + 3. A cancer's aggressiveness is related to the percentage of cancer that is grade 4 or 5. So how the two numbers are added together is important.

My discussions with Dr. Smith didn't give me many answers. He didn't know what caused the prostate cancer in my particular case. He knew of nothing that I had done in the past to increase my chances of this type of cancer. I didn't smoke and drank only on an occasional basis, mostly weekends. There was not a history of prostate cancer in my genes—my father at that time was eighty-six years old, and he did not have it. So the answer was to move forward with the next steps.

Chapter 4

Tests Done Prior to the Operation

There were several options to discuss involving what to do with this type of cancer. However, Dr. Smith wanted to rule out any other cancer in my body before we decided on a plan to approach.

First, he authorized a whole-body bone scan. A whole-body bone scan is used to detect whether the prostate cancer has spread. The spine and other bones are among the most common locations for the spread of prostate cancer. I had to call the nuclear medicine department of the large Chicagoland hospital to schedule this appointment. My insurance company required pre-certification and pre-approval for this service, which was provided by Dr. Smith. The whole-body bone scan procedure was scheduled for Thursday, April 3, 2003.

This procedure takes about five hours. There is no prep for this procedure. First, you come in for an IV injection of a radioactive tracer into your vein. Then the doctor suggests you go off, wait for two to four hours. The time is needed for the tracer to localize or be absorbed into your bones. The amount of radiation used in this test is small and well within limits, which is safe.

I hung around the local Corner Bakery, reading the newspaper and attempting to do some work for the four hours. Then you come back to the doctor's office, where you are first asked to empty your bladder so the pelvic and hip bones show up clearly. Then they begin the scan, which takes an hour and a half. You have to lie very still on a large flat table, and a total body image of your skeleton is taken.

It is very cold in the procedure area, and you are left alone while the machine completes the scan. The purpose of the procedure is to assess for skeletal metastases—cancer in the bones if you will. The results of the scan of my whole body noted degenerative changes, most prominent in the shoulders, wrists, ankles, and feet. There was more discussion about arthritic changes in my body. In summary, the whole-body bone scan demonstrated arthritic changes. There was no definite scintigraphic evidence of skeletal metastases. In other words, I did not have any cancer in my bones. What a relief.

Next, Dr. Smith authorized a CT of my chest (with and without contrast), a CT of my abdomen (with contrast), and a CT of my pelvis (with contrast). CT scans or CAT (computerized axial tomography scan) is a technique of evaluating the internal organs of the body with computerized x-ray pictures. For these procedures, I had to call the large medical hospital foundation's computed tomography department and make a reservation. Once again, my insurance required pre-certification and pre-registration, which was provided by Dr. Smith's office. These procedures took place on Wednesday, February 12, 2003.

All three tests took place at the same time. I had to be on a clear liquid diet for six hours before the procedure, nothing carbonated. These tests were rather quick in total time, taking a total of one hour and forty minutes. I arrived at the doctor's office and was asked to change. I was also given two large bottles of barium to drink. The nurse put an IV into my arm, which would make it easy to give me a shot of the dye or contrast at the appropriate time. I drank the first bottle of barium, nasty stuff, in half an hour. I was able to finish about three-quarters of the second bottle in the next half hour. It got worse trying to get this stuff down. It was thick and very sweet with a bad aftertaste.

The nurse then called me in for the actual tests. I was put into a tubelike machine and, once again, had to lie very still for twenty minutes. Inside the tubelike machine is another machine that revolves around you and generates a series of pictures. The computer then translates this information into pictures that look like cross sections of your body. It is pretty cool and the best way to look at your organs without surgery. First, I was run through the machine without the contrast or dye. Then they pulled me out of the tube and shot the dye into the IV in my arm, and plugged me back into the tube, this time with the dye. A machine within the tube took pictures of my chest, abdomen, and pelvis both times—without and with the dye. The dye is warm when it is inserted into your arm. It gave me an iron taste in my mouth and an iron smell in my nostrils. A warm sensation also felt like coming out of my anus; however, nothing came out.

This entire technique is called a helical CT of the chest, abdomen, and pelvis performed with the use of IV and oral contrast. A computed tomography (CT) scan is a special way of looking at the inside of your body. The images it produces are cross-sectional planes taken from a part of your body, much like slices taken out of a loaf of bread. The CT test is done in the radiology (x-ray) department at the large hospital.

Once again, the results were overwhelmingly positive. My cardiac (heart) size was normal. There were no pleural or pericardial effusions in my chest. There was no mediastinal or hilar lymphadenopathy, and there was no auxiliary lymphadenopathy. My lung windows demonstrated no pulmonary masses, nodules, or focal areas of consolidation. My lung base was clear. My bone windows demonstrated no evidence of osseous metastasis disease.

The results of the CT of my abdomen were that my liver, spleen, pancreas, adrenal glands, and both kidneys were unremarkable in appearance (which is good). There was no abdominal free fluid or any lymphadenopathy. There was no evidence of metastatic disease to my upper abdomen.

The results of the CT of my pelvis were that there was no pelvic free fluid or lymphadenopathy present. There were no pelvic masses. There was no evidence of metastatic disease to the pelvis.

In short, there was no evidence of metastatic disease in my chest, abdomen, or pelvis. These two major tests determined that I did not have any other cancer in my body.

The next step, according to Dr. Smith, was to determine if I was strong enough to handle a major operation. He authorized a stress echocardiogram.

Chapter 5

Stress Echocardiogram

I called the hospital ahead of time for my stress echocardiogram. The procedure was scheduled for the morning of Wednesday, April 16, 2003. I knew I was missing a lot of work, and I needed to attend an all-hands meeting back at one of my company's main facilities later in the day. I wanted to know if the hospital had an area where I could shower after the stress test. The receptionist put me on hold for several minutes and then responded, "Yes, we do," when she returned.

I arrive for my stress test dressed in my normal work attire, which is a suit and tie. I changed into my running clothes in the locker area that I was directed to by the attending nurse and proceeded to the area for the stress test. This was a pretty simple test for me, but I see where it could be hard for some people. I had been exercising for the past year and was in arguably the best shape of my life. The stress test, as it was explained to me, was basically hooking me up to a machine, registering my heart rate and blood pressure, and having me run on a treadmill. Attachments were stuck to my chest with small suction cups. I have a fairly hairy chest, and the nurse had to shave my chest in the areas where the suction cups were to be installed so they would stick to my skin.

Then I started walking on the treadmill. The treadmill started at a very slow speed which was increased every two minutes or so. For an additional challenge, the treadmill increased in incline each time the speed was increased. It started out slow and flat, but by twenty minutes, it was up to a good pace, and I was running hard and had

WILLIAM J. VOLLER, JR.

to hold on to the bar on the front of the treadmill because the incline was so steep.

There were three nurses in the room administering the stress test to me. After watching me run for a few minutes, they started asking me questions about my exercise routine. Once they discovered that I was a daily runner and swimmer, the head nurse called for two additional resources (nurses). In order for the echocardiogram to work, the patient's heart rate has to be at a high level, and it must maintain that level for some time for the echocardiograph to register correct information. The problem with runners is that after they stop running, their bodies recover very quickly, and their heart rate drops fast.

It took about twenty minutes on the treadmill for me to reach the heart rate level required. During that time, the five-person nurse team was preparing for the steps they would need to take to get me off of the treadmill and to have the echocardiograph register correctly. They were explaining this process to me while I was running. They indicated that typically they see older people taking this test. At best, these older people put on a pair of running shoes or tennis shoes that they own. But they usually wear street clothes. And they usually last less than five minutes on the treadmill. They just step off the treadmill and are breathing so hard after five minutes that the test is completed very easily.

In my case, when the nurses believed that my heart rate and blood pressure was suitably high enough, they would have to quickly lift me off of the treadmill and place me down on the table, all the while inserting the echocardiogram device under my ribs on my left side by my heart so they could complete the test before my body started to recover and my heart rate dropped. They had some large women there, and at the right time, they lifted me off of the treadmill and inserted the device in my left side, all the while reminding me not to try to breathe so the test could be completed successfully. I am sure it was a rather comical sight, these nurses picking up this sweaty man and throwing him on the table, all while yelling at him to hold his breath. All I wanted to do was to gulp for air.

26

The nurses indicated that they had not had anyone like me there for a long time. The results of my stress echocardiogram were excellent.

But that was not the end of the story.

I went back to my locker, damp and sweaty. I needed a shower. I asked the nurse where I could find one. She looked back at me quizzically—I knew I was in trouble. Since this team usually had older patients taking the stress test who usually took the test in their street clothes, they didn't use a shower. In fact, it was such a long time since the patient shower area had been used that it had become a shortcut walkway between the two main work areas on the floor. Doctors and nurses used this shortcut all day long. The nurses quickly set it up for me, shutting the doors and giving me some privacy. However, that didn't last. As soon as I started showering, doctors and nurses opened the doors and walked through the shower area, looking at me as if I was from Mars. I soaped up and rinsed off as quickly as possible, but I am sure that at least twenty people came through that area while I was showering. I am not sure who was more embarrassed, me or the doctors and nurses? Everyone laughed and excused themselves as they walked through the area, but I felt rather embarrassed.

I dressed quickly and made it back to work in time for the meeting, but I had to laugh at the experiences I had that morning—from the stress test to the shower—both were funny and unique to me.

Part 2

(May, June, July 2003)

Chapter 6

Options to Review / Decisions to Be Made

Dr. Smith was ready to discuss the options with me. I had passed the tests without any problem, and my body was significantly strong enough to handle major surgery if necessary.

There were more options than I thought. Basically, there are five of them. We discussed them all in detail. By we, I mean Dr. Smith, Cory, and me. It was a difficult morning.

The first option is called watchful waiting. It is basically an option that older men may select. It means coming to the doctor on a regular basis and taking a regular PSA test. Prostate cancer is rather slow-growing, and older men may feel more comfortable with this. It is an active program of regular monitoring of cancer. What it does *not* mean is to go home and never return for follow-up exams and PSA blood tests. Very simply, this option is a non-active treatment for cancer. As I said, this is best suited for men in their seventies and eighties with a limited long-term life expectancy. It could also be a suitable option for men in their sixties and early seventies who have also been diagnosed with other potentially life-threatening health problems. I guess you should ask yourself, "What is going to get me first?" Is it prostate cancer or something else? On one hand, I think most people would agree to avoid unnecessary treatment and potential risks. On the other hand, it is sad if a person dies from treatable prostate cancer. This could happen if the person lives longer than expected. If you live long enough, untreated cancer will kill you.

The second option is radical prostatectomy. This is the most invasive option and means surgery. It is a major operation. However, it removes cancer from the body. This is the option I chose. I wanted the cancer out. I wanted it out of my body before it had a chance to spread to other organs. The best candidate for this option is a younger man. There are three criteria that you should look at when considering this option. The prostate cancer should be confined to the prostate itself, which the whole-body bone scan and the three CT scans that I completed fully demonstrated. The patient should be able to safely undergo this operation requiring general anesthesia, which I had proven by my excellent score on the echocardiography test. And finally, the patient should have a life expectancy long enough to see the benefits of the surgery. My father was eighty-five years old at the time of my surgery. He was still alive ten years later, at the age of ninety-five. As a side note, you should know that he had been ultimately diagnosed with prostate cancer. He selected the *watchful waiting* option.

The third option is a form of radiation therapy, either external beam/IMRT or radioactive seeds. The external beam and IMRT (intensity-modulated radiation therapy) options use radiation in highly focused and computer-generated beams to the prostate. The beams of high-energy radiation are focused from outside of the body onto the targeted prostate or other target areas. There is no surgery with this option. One should really discuss this option with your doctor to fully comprehend the total advantages and disadvantages. Radiation takes a long time—almost a full seven weeks on a Monday through Friday basis to be successful. Many men experience some form of either bladder or rectum irritation during the seven-week process, sometimes both. Most experts agree that radiation therapy is as effective as radical prostatectomy for the first seven to ten years after the treatment. There is some debate about long-term results. I will discuss this option in more detail later in this book.

The second option of radiation is radioactive seed implants. This option sounded interesting to me, and I spent a great deal of time thinking about it. What is it? How does it work? During this process, tiny rice-sized pellets, which have been specially treated to be radioactive, are inserted into the prostate. The radiation they release into the prostate kills the adjacent cancer cells. Pellets can be energized with various amounts of radiation so a radiation therapist can decide how many seeds are needed and what dose each seed should contain. However, experts, in general, agree that men with high-grade cancer (PSA of 10 or better) or with a Gleason score of 7 or above or men with a large prostate are more likely to fail this method. So the best candidates are men with small amounts of low-grade cancer, with a PSA of less than 10, and with small prostates. This ruled me out with my Gleason score of 7 on the right side of my prostate.

The number of seeds placed in the prostate varies, as I stated. It could range from forty to one hundred fifty, with the average being about eighty. It takes about one and one-half to two hours to insert the seeds. The process is done through the skin of the perineum, which is just under the scrotum in front of the anus. The patient obviously needs to be under anesthesia during the process, either localized or general, where you are put to sleep. Usually, men are in the hospital overnight for this procedure and go home the next day.

You will have to wait several months, if not a year, to fully realize the results of the seed radiation on your PSA score. It should go down gradually. Dr. Smith did explain to me the one major disadvantage of this surgery. He stated that the radiation does damage the surrounding organs in the body. And if the PSA does not go down, a radical prostatectomy is very difficult, if not impossible, to do.

The fourth option is destructive therapies. The two major ones are cryotherapy (or freezing of the prostate gland) and HIFU. Cryotherapy is the controlled freezing of the prostate gland for cancer treatment. The intent is to kill the cancer cells. During this procedure, the prostate tissue is frozen. Under anesthesia, special probes are placed throughout the prostate. Liquid nitrogen or Argon gas is circulated through the probes. This freezes the tissue of the prostate. The goal is to create a large ice ball big enough to kill cancer. One major issue is that up to 80 percent or more of the men who have undergone this procedure have complained about impotence afterward. The risk of impotence depends upon how aggressively the doctor freezes the prostate tissues. This procedure works best for those men whose prostate is on the smaller size, about forty grams or less in size.

HIFU (High-Intensity Focused Ultrasound) is something new. It was not available as an option when I was selecting which option to use. High-energy ultrasound waves are focused through a rectal probe into the prostate. This ultrasound energy is then directed into the prostate under real-time guidance. This energy is converted into heat within the meat of the prostate, effectively "cooking" the prostate tissues and thus killing cancer. This procedure takes about one to three hours. HIFU appears to be best used as initial therapy for localized prostate cancer or to treat the prostate for rising PSA after radiation failure.

The last or fifth option is hormonal therapy. This could include monthly hormone injections or removal of the testicles or chemotherapy. Generally, what happens with hormonal therapy is that the hormone is removed from the body during treatment because prostate cancer is hormone-sensitive. The hormone testosterone actually stimulates prostate cancer growth. When the hormone is removed from the body, cancer usually stops growing and may go into a dormant or hibernation stage. The best candidate for this type of treatment is a man whose prostate cancer disease has shown signs of progression even after radiation or surgery. This is usually the primary treatment for older men when they want to do something more than just *watchful waiting*, but the option of radiation or surgery is just too much to handle or not appropriate.

There you have it, the options Dr. Smith, Cory, and I discussed. It actually was more than a bit overwhelming and technical. My head was spinning from all of the information. What do I do? Which is the right option? The decision was mine to make. Cory and I drove home in silence; I was doing some serious thinking the whole way.

Chapter 7

Life Source Blood Donation and Additional Discussions

Cory and I had many conversations during the following days. Ultimately, I had to do what I felt was right for my body. But I wanted to make sure that Cory was comfortable with my decision. The decision was mine to make, but Cory had a huge interest and was really invested in the process and outcome. I knew I wanted the cancer out. I didn't want anything in my body that could spread to other organs and tissues. For me, the only answer was the radical prostatectomy.

Cory and I talked about this option as well as the others. We finally agreed, and I contacted Dr. Smith with our decision. He was pleased and agreed with my option selection. We now were in a stage Dr. Smith called the *window of opportunity*. This can be defined as between the point where the cancer is confirmed with a diagnosis and when it starts to spread.

We needed to actively move forward with a plan prior to the point where cancer begins to spread. Prostate cancer is very slow-growing and may have been in my body for several years or decades, but that window stays open for only a short period of time.

We initially made plans to schedule the surgery for July of 2003. In the meantime, Dr. Smith wanted me to start storing my blood to use during or after the surgery. This process was the same as any blood donation process anyone would do for donation purposes or profit. For me, it was a potential lifesaving issue. The best blood to get during surgery is your own. It has the best chances of being accepted by your body.

This was a two-week process—beginning on June 23 and ending on July 7, 2003. After the initial meeting, I would drive to the local blood bank in my area several times per week, and they would remove some of my blood. It was then stored for use during my surgery. I was not aware of this process and was pleasantly surprised that it was available. It is somewhat ghoulish in nature; people are lying on tables throughout the space of this facility, and their blood is being removed. About a hundred feet away is a major grocery store; people are moving back and forth in front of the windows to the facility. I know I passed by this blood bank location hundreds of times without really knowing what went on inside. The process was quick and painless. Once it was complete, I had an amount of my blood available, if needed, for the surgery.

Soon after completing my blood collection and storage activity, Cory and I met with a nurse in the urology department to discuss a few very important topics—one of which was sex after this type of invasive surgery. Many things can happen during the surgery, but the nurse assured us that our sex life should continue as strong as it was before the operation. Cory and I were fairly healthy adults who were in love with one another—even after twenty-five years of marriage. We had sex between two and three times per week. This frank discussion with the nurse led us to believe that a healthy sex life prior to the surgery will assist in making sure that a similar sex life could be continued after surgery.

Finally, we also discussed the possibility of incontinence or the control of urine after this type of operation. One of the prostate's main functions for men is to control their urine flow. Men are born with this organ. The prostate, along with a combination of other organs and muscles, assisted in the control of the flow of our urine, stopping it when needed and making sure that urine flow did not leak.

When the prostate is removed from the base of the bladder, some damage can occur to the urinary sphincter, which holds the urine naturally. This results in incontinence—a future state no man looks forward to. Actually, the nurse informed me of a very simple set of exercises called *pelvic floor muscle exercises*. This is a series of quick muscular tightening actions, which strengthen the pelvic muscles. Women have used these muscles since they were born to assist in urine control. Men have relied on our prostates. She suggested doing these exercises frequently before the operation to make sure that my muscles were ready after the operation. I was to do them for five minutes every hour that I was awake—really not a big deal. I was going to do anything to make sure that I didn't have a urine flow control problem after my surgery. One problem is, you don't really know how good you are doing since your prostate was still in place, and that took care of all potential leakage issues.

Actually, Cory and I left this meeting in a much better frame of mind than after our last meeting with Dr. Smith. I was confident that we would continue our normal sex pattern, even after the surgery, and I knew I was going to be able to control my urine after the surgery.

On to surgery!

Part 3

(August 2003)

Chapter 8

Radical Retropubic Prostatectomy Surgery

As I stated earlier, the operation was scheduled for mid-July of 2003. One day, early in July, Dr. Smith called me and asked about moving the surgery a little bit. Dr. Smith had scheduled a short vacation, and he was looking forward to it.

Actually, I informed Dr. Smith that I had planned a nice vacation in the late July / early August period on Hilton Head Island with the entire family after the operation. Dr. Smith said that it would be best if I enjoyed my vacation before the surgery. Prostate cancer is a very slow-growing cancer, and he was confident that my *window of opportunity* would still be open, even after I returned from vacation. We agreed to schedule the surgery for Wednesday, August 13, 2003. Now both of us could enjoy our vacations prior to the surgery.

Our family had a great time on Hilton Head Island. We golfed and enjoyed the sand, surf, food, and culture of the island. This was not our first trip to Hilton Head, so we exactly knew what we wanted to do and where to go to get it. Cory and I had some very romantic dinners alone. The food and drinks were fabulous. I was well-rested and prepared for the future when I returned home to Illinois.

Operation Day—August 13, 2003. Dr. Smith is a bit of a control nut. He wants everything to be perfect. His preparation is flawless, and his demand for his patients to be as prepared as possible is legendary.

The evening before the surgery, I had to begin the cleansing process. This process is done at home and is initiated by consuming a bad-tasting fluid, which caused me to go to the washroom multiple times. I believe it is the same prep process that someone goes through for a colonoscopy. Let me assure you; it is complete. In a few hours, I was empty and very clean. However, I was starving, and my stomach was very upset. I went to bed and tried to get some sleep.

The next day before I left home, Dr. Smith wanted me to have an enema just to make sure I was clean. And if that was not enough, I had another enema administered to me right after I checked in to the hospital by a beautiful blond young attendant. I've got to admit; I was somewhat embarrassed. I was empty down there, and I knew I was clean, that is for sure!

Cory and I drove downtown together early in the morning. The large hospital has a very nice practice in which they allow the spouses of the patients to stay in the rooms with them during their recovery. Cory had packed a small overnight bag. I had packed a few things also—a toothbrush, hairbrush, pajamas, a thin housecoat, and house slippers.

My two sons joined us also. Cory was crying; I was trying to keep a strong face. However, when the young blond attendant came to give me the enema, both boys laughed, and my composure broke; I laughed with them.

Soon after the last enema, Dr. Smith came in to greet me. Several other doctors and nurses also made their introductions. They began to prepare me for the operation. I had IVs placed into the veins of my arm. I had suction cups taped to my chest. White tape was everywhere, holding things into place. I was told to get ready. I said my goodbyes to my wife and sons, and I was wheeled into the operating room. This is a huge hospital. It takes a long time to get from one end of the hospital to the other, plus it is a multistory complex, so there are elevators to enter and leave. Moving is a big process like a parade. The operating room was big and cold—very cold with subdued lighting. I especially noted that the ceiling was high. Nurses brought in warm blankets and tucked them all around me to keep me warm. In a matter of minutes, the anesthetic was administered, and I was asleep.

Chapter 9

Recovery in the Hospital

I woke up. Well, I made it. I am alive.

I opened my eyes, and I realized that I was in a large recovery room being monitored and supervised by several nurses. I didn't feel too bad. I felt very warm and snug. I closed my eyes again and just waited for a few moments.

Soon I decided that it was time to try to move around, just slightly. What a mistake! Man, did that hurt. *Wow*! I was suddenly in a great deal of pain right in the area where the surgery took place. I could barely raise my hand to get the nurse's attention. The nurse flew to my side and welcomed me back. She asked how I was feeling; I could barely respond; the pain was so sharp.

The nurse shot a needle full of something into one of the IVs in my arm, and soon I felt no pain.

The nurse called up to my room to notify them that I was awake and that I would be transferred to their care in the near future. An aide was assigned to this duty. My aide must have been a "Romeo." He knew everyone in the hospital and stopped on several occasions to talk to others (young ladies) while he was making his way to my recovery room. I was on a flat gurney and could not see who he was talking to, but I could hear the conversations, and he certainly knew what he was doing.

Finally, I arrived at my room. Cory was still crying, and my son Bradley had stayed with her during the procedure. I greeted both of them with a smile. Cory said that I looked "like hell." It had taken several hours for the operation and my recovery, but I was told that everything went "fine." One of the first things my room attendants wanted me to do, believe it or not, was to walk. I was in no mood to move at all. In fact, all I wanted to do was sleep. But the attendants had told Cory that the healing process would go quicker if I walked. The body has to get back to normal, they told her.

Cory knew it was going to be difficult to get me to move, so she whispered in my ear that the hospital was having pizza for lunch that day, and I could get a few slices, if I made a strong attempt at walking.

She was right; that did it. I was hungry from the night before, and the pizza sounded great to me. Reluctantly, I agreed to the walk. Now, this was no ordinary stroll around the room for a few feet. *No.* This was a hike. I walked two times around the entire floor. I had an army surrounding me. Cory was holding one of my hands. I had the portable IV unit in my other arm. However, the joke was on me. No pizza. In fact, on day one after the surgery, all you can have is a clear liquid diet.

As I stated earlier, the hospital room that I was assigned allowed Cory to stay with me during my entire hospital stay. She had a small area next to me set up as a bed, and she could use the cafeteria for food. It was very convenient.

The first night in the hospital after the operation, I was in a great deal of pain. I had refused any pain medicine, trying to be a "macho man." Cory told me that I should take the meds. Naturally, I refused. What an idiot!

I could not get to sleep, and finally, as soon as I did, it seemed that the nurses would rush into the room, taking my temperature and checking the drain from the surgery and the urine bag. I did discover what was causing me so much pain. My doctor, Dr. Smith, was considered "old school." At the end of the operation, he inserted a small stitch into the head of my penis to hold the catheter in place. What a guy! About halfway through the night, I finally relented and asked for some medication to help with the pain. Whatever they gave me worked perfectly. I was asleep in no time.

The surgery resulted in a small vertical incision between my belly button and my penis, about 2.5 to 3.0 inches in length. A small clear plastic drain tube had been inserted in this incision to allow for run-off of fluids from the wound. This was in addition to the catheter from my penis. The nurses would be required to check these two drip lines to make sure they were operating correctly. The drain from the incision had to dry before you were allowed to leave the hospital.

On the days immediately following the surgery, once you can tolerate clear liquids, you can begin receiving solid foods. There will be an emphasis on two things: breathing deeply and coughing every hour while you are awake and walking at least two to three times per day.

I recovered quickly and was scheduled to leave the hospital after three days, which was normal. You all know the drill; you have to move your bowels before they allow you to leave the hospital. You are given a stool softener to assist you in the process. I completed that requirement and was getting ready to go home. We were all in a good mood.

The last thing that had to be completed was a short course by the nurse, instructing me on how to deal with my catheter as well as how to change and care for the urine collection bags. The hospital provided me with two types of bags for the catheter: one style I could attach to my leg, allowing me to be mobile. The second type was used during sleep-times and could be attached to my bed called a drainage bag.

There was an on-off button that allowed me to switch from drainage bag mode to the mobile leg mode and back again. The nurse showed me how to operate the button and actually had me do it by myself before she left the room. Now I was all set to go home. Yeah!

Part 4

(August, September,
October 2003)

Chapter 10

Life and Results After Surgery

On the way home, my bladder began to feel full. It takes about an hour to drive to Wheaton from the large hospital in Chicago, and that is in light traffic. During the trip, I felt more and more uncomfortable. I noticed that the mobile leg bag did not seem to have any urine in it but not having worn a "mobile unit" before, I did not know how much urine should be in it. All I knew was that I felt like I was going to explode.

I was in a lot of pain, and Cory knew it. She could tell in my eyes, and she could tell by the tone of my voice. I didn't know what was wrong. We were home only about half an hour when we decided to go to the local hospital near Wheaton to find out what was wrong. Cory rushed through traffic. I could barely breathe; I was in so much pain. I was rushed into the emergency ward of the hospital. Cory explained that I had just returned home from prostate cancer surgery, and the doctor looked me over and fiddled with the on-off button. The urine came rushing into the bag, and I immediately felt relieved. All the pressure was off, and I could begin to think again. What a miserable experience!

We returned home, and Cory and I got back to some sort of normal while I was healing at home. I transferred from mobile leg bag catheter mode to permanent drainage bag mode every evening before I went to bed and then back to mobile leg mode when I woke up each morning. The mobile catheter was very convenient.

It allowed me to walk about the house and even go outside (wearing long pants).

You can shower once you are home; just keep the area of the surgery as dry as possible. The incision healed quickly and was soon closed shut.

After a few weeks, I was instructed to have the catheter removed. All during this time and actually before operation, I was doing the pelvic floor muscle exercises.

Men are spoiled. They never have to do pelvic floor muscle exercises unless they have their prostate removed. As I stated earlier, the prostate stops bladder leaks. But now that my prostate was gone, I was leaking like crazy. The catheter didn't help. It allowed the urine to flow freely; that was its intent. But now, with my prostate removed and the catheter removed, I was on my own. I had to do pelvic floor muscle exercises and do them religiously. You just have to exercise them internally as much as you can. The pelvic floor maintains the urine in the bladder and prevents leakage. It relaxes during normal urination and allows urine to flow freely.

It was great to get rid of the catheter. I was free and normal, but I did have slight urine leakage, even after doing the pelvic floor exercises.

After ten days or so, I was able to control my urine leaks. Of course, if I laughed hard or sneezed hard, I still had minor leakage. I am not proud of it, but I had to wear an adult diaper for a short amount of time. Just to make sure there were no minor disasters. Of course, I was at home most of the time so any accidents could be taken care of immediately.

I went back to work in a few weeks and continued with my life as if nothing had happened.

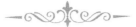

Chapter 11

Sex After Surgery
Premade Injections and the
Pharmacological Erection Program

There was a little problem.

While I had no interest in sex immediately after the surgery, I was becoming a little frisky after a few weeks. The problem was, I could not get an erection. Discussions with the doctor and nurse prior to the surgery assured me that sex was going to continue after the surgery, but with me, nothing happened. I just couldn't get an erection. I was shocked, and so was my wife.

We made an appointment to see the doctor and asked him what was going on. Doctor Smith informed us that during the surgery, he had noticed that the nerves on one side of my penis did not look correct to him, so he removed them. I still had these nerves on the other side of my penis. The problem is that you need both sets of nerves to achieve a full erection. I was not told of this possible outcome prior to the operation, nor was I informed that the nerves were removed after the operation.

To say that we (my wife and I) were pissed was an understatement. I was livid. What was the planned solution?

We discussed things with the doctor, and he prescribed the normal medications—I had prescriptions to both Viagra and Cialis. I tried both to no avail. Neither one worked to give me an erection. After I took either of them, all that happened to me was that I saw a rainbow effect around objects, especially in strong sunlight in rooms. I don't know about you, but to me, this was a *big* problem. Just as big of a problem as cancer had been.

What was I going to do? I was fifty-one years old, and I could not get an erection? That was unheard of.

We had more discussions and meetings with Dr. Smith. He brought in a urology clinical neurological specialist from the hospital for consultation. Dr. Smith had worked with this individual before on patients similar to me. Several options were discussed and reviewed:

1. Obviously, the easiest and simplest solution was the pills—either Viagra or Cialis, if they worked. In my case, they did not work. Strike out this option.
2. Have another operation to install a pump-type device into the penis. This would allow you to pump up your penis prior to insertion for sex. This just didn't seem like a good solution to me. It required another operation, and at that time, I was quite done with operations, especially down there!
3. Premade injections. This option involved giving yourself a shot in the penis with a special prescribed amount of fluid. The chemicals in the fluid would surge through the penis and make it erect. It would last for some time, and then the erection would go down, just like it would normally after sex.
4. Individually prescribed shots similar to the premade system but more clearly defined specifically to suit your needs and requirements for an erection.

We had tried the first option without success. To be honest with you, the second option was just not appealing to me. That left the last two options. I was getting desperate. Things were not looking favorable for me. Would I ever get an erection again?

Cory and I tried the third option—special premade injections. I am not sure how these were developed, but they were shipped to me via the mail in prefilled amounts. This was a big procedure. I had to administer a shot into my penis by myself. I was not a huge fan of shots in the first place, and giving yourself a shot in the most sensitive area of a man's body was not a pleasant thought.

They arrived, and I tried them. The procedure insists upon a great deal of cleanliness. Washing your hands several times during the process, wiping alcohol swabs over the area prior to and after insertion was required. The injection site is under the head of the penis, along either side. Once the needle is injected, you must then inject the medication into the penis.

However, we quickly found out that the premade injections did not work as expected. They come all prepackaged, so I did not have to put the medicine into the syringe, but the dosage just did not work out for me.

Finally, after much frustration and worry, we tried the individually prescribed shots.

Let me tell you what I had to go through for these shots. First, they had to get the right dosage of the medicine. They landed on a tri-mix solution containing PGE-1, phentolamine and papaverine. Prior to inserting this solution into my penis by myself, I had to go through the process with a male sex specialist. I had to prove to him that I knew how to do it right. We started off with me giving the injection to a rubber penis. Humorous but good for training and preparation. Next, I had to do it to myself while the specialist watched. I was not looking forward to that.

I am somewhat of a modest introvert. I was not one to show my erection to anyone besides my wife. Now I had to go through the set of instructions with a male "observer."

First, you have to prepare the shot. Wash your hands thoroughly. Clean the top of the vial with an alcohol wipe. Remove the plastic cover from the needle and the plastic cover of the plunger. Draw back the empty syringe and pull the plunger down to the dosage mark to fill with air, shoot air into the vile. Pull back the plunger, allowing the syringe to fill with the tri-mix beyond the recommended amount of dosage. Then flick the syringe with your fingers to remove any bubbles and get the air to the top of the syringe, holding the needle upright. Shoot some tri-mix medication back into the vial so you only have the correct dosage amount of tri-mix in the syringe. Then place the cap back on the top of the needle and set it down.

Next, you wash your hands again. Sit down. Take an alcohol wipe and wipe the area on your penis when you intend to shoot in the tri-mix solution. Place the needle on the skin of the penis and pierce through the skin until the needle is in the flesh up the hub. Push the plunger to empty the tri-mix medication into your penis. This part really smarts! The tip of my penis usually feels mild pain and a slight "burning" sensation while this is happening. Remove the injection from the penis and wipe off the pierced area of your penis with an alcohol wipe.

Within a short amount of time, you have an erection. And a pretty good one. It lasts for a while. In fact, if it lasts over four hours, you are instructed to go immediately to an emergency room. My erections last a while now but never long enough to require emergency room trips.

Well, I passed the first test with my "observer," and I was on my own. I have been giving myself shots now for the past sixteen years, the process still works. However, I must admit that it takes some of the spontaneity out of the sexual encounter. You have to rotate the sites of the shot as well as the sides of the penis you use so one side of the penis isn't overly used. You should not inject yourself more than once in a twenty-four-hour period. They recommend using the tri-mix medication about two times a week at most. That has been the way we have sex now ever since my operation in 2003.

Part 5

(Late 2003, 2004, 2005, and 2006)

Chapter 12

May Be a Lab Error

After my operation and recovery in 2003, I began a series of visits with Dr. Smith on a regular basis just to perform a PSA test and see the results. These were quick visits, just a simple blood test, and I was back on the street. The first of these tests occurred on August 25, 2003, twelve days after the surgery. The note I received from Dr. Smith on August 28, 2003, after he reviewed the data, was as follows, "PSA is 0.5. Coming down nicely. Should be 0.0 by next visit."

The next visit was November 12, 2003. Once again, a simple blood test to obtain a PSA score. The result of this PSA was 0.0. Dr. Smith was elated and sent a statement to me dated November 23, 2003, which was "perfect." This was truly a fantastic thanksgiving present from God. What a relief to have a 0.0 PSA score. I was truly "cancer-free." Okay, now we had to set up additional return visits. Another PSA test was scheduled for six months in the future, with an MD exam scheduled in one year.

I had the next PSA test on August 6, 2004. Once again, the results were 0.0. Dr. Smith stated that "the PSA is undetectable in this patient. Please relay the good news." Once again, I had a sigh of relief, and I was building up confidence that this was all behind me and that I could begin to go forward with my life. I was cancer-free for one full year!

My next PSA test was scheduled for one whole year later, on Thursday, August 4, 2005. It was a "nurse appointment," just to draw blood. What could go wrong? However, just when I was just getting comfortable, this PSA score came back as 0.1. It went up. Boy, things went racing through my mind. How could this be? What is going on? Is this normal? The comment I received from Dr. Smith was, "He thinks this is just a lab error. Have the test repeated in two to three months."

That was comforting. Now I had to wait three months before I found out what was going on. I had to go to work every day. I had to be a husband, father, provider and act like nothing was happening or nothing was going to interfere with my "regular" life. Right, like I could do that.

The follow-up PSA test was scheduled for October 5, 2005. The PSA drawn on that date was 0.2. Once again, the PSA score was going up! It was not a "lab error," but the fact was, I still had prostate cancer!

Great. I felt terrible. Now what! What were the next steps?

Chapter 13

Tests Prior to Radiation

Dr. Smith, in his comforting, professional way, was, as usual, very black and white. By the book. He termed my condition a biochemical relapse of prostate cancer. First thing he wanted done was for me to undergo CT scans of the chest, abdomen, and pelvis, without and with infusion, a bone scan, and a ProstaScint scan. Once I complete these tests, I should schedule an appointment with him to go over the results and determine the next steps. He did discuss what this meant. He stated that approximately 20 percent of men who have prostate surgery have follow-up positive PSA scores.

He believed that there were microscopic prostate tumor cells that remained in the area of the prostate after the surgery. The surgery caused them to become dormant. However, in the two years since the surgery, these cells had reawakened and caused this increase in PSA. He did not feel that this was in any way life-threatening. He believed that it was not imminent. This was somewhat comforting to me. But not really. I thought I had this cancer thing behind me. Now it was right up in my face again. Let me tell you, it is not easy to live a regular life and enjoy regular things when this is hanging over your head.

The three CT scans of the chest, abdomen, and pelvis were scheduled for Tuesday, October 25, 2005. They were held at the large hospital's computed tomography center. These tests were done with and without dye infusion. The prep was no fluids for six hours prior to the tests.

The bone scan was done the following week, Tuesday, November 1, 2005, at the nuclear medicine department within the hospital. There was no prep for this exam. Bone scans take some time. You arrive at the hospital. They check you in and register. Then they give you a shot and have some discussion with you. Then they tell you to leave and return in approximately two hours. They expect you to eat somewhat lightly during the two-hour time frame. There was a total of four tests: the pelvis area, a whole-body scan, hands above your head for the chest and hands on top of the stomach, head to the left, and head to the right. The scans took a total of about one hour. You kept your clothes on during these tests; no jewelry or metal allowed.

The ProstaScint exam is a two-day test. Day one was scheduled for Friday, November 4, 2005, once again, at the nuclear medicine department of the hospital. The prep was nothing to eat or drink after midnight the night before. Similar to the bone scan, this test has multiple steps. The patient checks in and is registered, then the patient receives an injection of In-111 ProstaScint, a radioactive pharmaceutical. It can stay in your body for up to a month after injection. Afterward, I received a letter from the hospital for me to use if I traveled, alerting whoever was concerned about the possibility that radiation monitoring devices may detect radiation within my body.

After getting the injection, I was sent out for about an hour and a half to eat lightly. Once I returned, I was given several gowns to change into and then was told to lie flat on my back with my hands over my head for one hour, while they completed the tests.

Day two of the exam was Tuesday, November 8, 2005, again in the nuclear medicine department. The prep included taking *Dulcolax* for cleansing the night before right after dinner—two pills as well as abstaining from food and drink after midnight, the night before the exam. This is a long exam. It was a total of four tests; each one was one hour in length. Test one—hands above head. Test two—hands at side. Then they draw blood and have your hands above your head, and finally, they insert the blood back in and have the last test with your hands above your head.

Just a note about this procedure. This is done in the nuclear medicine area. Quite scary. They give you the shot while wearing a leaded apron. While you are going through the exam, no one else is in the room. The attendants peek in at you via a small window in the door every once in a while. Plus, the room is *cold*! I mean very cold! And the exam is *long*! You've got to stay perfectly still for the duration of the exam.

All of these tests were done to determine and eliminate any concern about cancer being in any of my other organs. These tests are called *restaging*, and the results were that they did not reveal overt/objective evidence of relapse.

Chapter 14

Expectant Management

I had two appointments with Dr. Smith after these tests. One on Wednesday, November 8, 2005, and the second on Monday, November 28, 2005. Dr. Smith explained to me that the results of these tests indicated that there was no definite evidence of metastatic disease elsewhere in my body.

It was decided that we would continue with *expectant management* for the time being. A return visit was planned for six months, and definite actions would take place if the PSA rose above 0.3 ng/mL.

My next appointment was scheduled for March 1, 2006. Once again, it included a PSA test. And, once again, my PSA score rose to 0.3 ng/mL. This started the restaging tests all over again.

The two-part ProstaScint exam was scheduled for Thursday, April 6, 2006, and Monday, April 10, 2006. The CT scans of the chest, abdomen, and pelvis, with and without dye, were scheduled for April 12, 2006. The bone scan was scheduled for April 18, 2006. On April 7, 2006, I received another letter from the hospital's radiation safety officer that indicated that I had received 6.2 mCi of In-111 ProstaScint, a radioactive pharmaceutical.

On April 10, 2006, Dr. Smith scheduled an appointment with me to discuss and make me seriously consider *hormone therapy*. Hormone therapy treatment requires taking pills for two weeks and shots for four months in order to reduce male hormone development. The issue is to impact libido and sexual desire. It also is used as a prelude to radiation around the area of the prostate. I was not real keen on this option.

On April 12, 2006, Dr. Smith's office reported to me that the CT scans did not reveal any obvious evidence of recurrent prostate cancer or cancer anywhere else. This was good news. The result of the bone scan was also negative. More good news.

The April 18, 2006, whole-body bone scan was compared to the prior whole-body bone scan study completed on November 1, 2005. The April 12 CT scans of the chest, abdomen, and pelvis with and without dye were compared to the October 25 CT of the same areas. The results were that there was no interval change in comparison to the prior study. Once again, it was decided to continue *expectant management* with a follow-up visit scheduled for June 1, 2006.

Obviously, a PSA test was completed on June 1, 2006, with the same results. No increase in PSA levels; however, the PSA remained 0.3 ng/mL. This was the second straight score of 0.3 ng/mL.

Now Dr. Smith was getting really aggressive and began scheduling other doctors for me to see to discuss hormone therapy and follow-up radiation. I spoke to Dr. Sue Blaha and Dr. Jim Doe MD from the hematology/oncology department of the large hospital on June 23, 2006. They both recommended radiation with androgen deprivation. More expectant management was advised with a follow-up appointment scheduled for around July 13, 2006, with Dr. Tony (oncologist) and Dr. Rey (radiation oncologist).

One interesting result of the blood test administered on June 1, 2006, was that my testosterone value was 3.23. The low level for a male of my age was 2.00, and the high level was 8.00. In my opinion, my score of 3.23 was on the low side. I wondered why was there such a push for me to enter into hormone therapy, which would reduce male hormone development? I started to think I needed a second opinion.

Another PSA test was done on July 20, 2006, with the same results. My PSA score was 0.3 ng/mL. This was the third score of 0.3 ng/mL (March 1, June 1, and July 20). The good news was that it was not increasing, but the bad news was that it was still there.

Part 6

(June Through
November 2006)

Chapter 15

Tattoos and Radiation

I next meet with doctors at the large hospital to continue discussions on the "next steps." One meeting involved getting two small dot tattoos on my body, one on either side on my hips. I was informed that these dots would be used to make sure that the radiation would be directed to the exact location every day. Dr. Smith was still pressing for hormonal therapy but also for beginning a daily regime of radiation for seven weeks.

At the time, I was working in the western suburbs of Chicago. I could take time off from work to address individual doctor and hospital visits, but daily visits were a whole other thing entirely. It took me about forty-five minutes to one hour to drive to Chicago for a doctor's visit. That is why I usually make these visits first thing in the morning. I could get downtown and have my appointment then, with a little bit of luck, be back in my office by noon.

Going to daily radiation in downtown Chicago would really impact my job. Especially since I was told that I could not pick the time of the day for the radiation. Mostly everyone has similar interests that I do, so time spots early in the day or late in the day were already taken.

I was in a bind.

I was sitting at home on Sunday, June 18, 2006, reading a Chicago newspaper. On Sundays, this newspaper includes a magazine section. This magazine was particularly focused on topics important to men since it was Father's Day weekend. One article that grabbed my attention on how a local television reporter had beat prostate cancer. In October of 2005, this television weekend's coanchor was told by his urologist that his prostate biopsy results came back positive for cancer. The article talked about how he went to a hospital in the western suburbs. Doctors there use TomoTherapy, which targets radiation on the cancerous area.

This sounded interesting to me. I read the complete article.

I contacted the hospital in the western suburbs on June 23, 2006. As I earlier mentioned, I was working in the western suburbs. This hospital in the western suburbs is very close to my work location. In fact, it is 2.8 miles away from my office, about a five-minute drive away. Perfect!

Based upon my June 23 telephone call to the hospital, I set up my first meeting with Dr. Mitch Strodel, the medical director of radiation oncology at the cancer care center of the hospital, for July 14, 2006.

This first meeting, besides sharing insurance and personal physical information, included an hour and a half consultation and Q and A with Dr. Strodel. It went great. Dr. Strodel was a young man who calmly answered all of my questions.

Based upon my conversation with Dr. Strodel, it was decided that I would begin a seven-week regime of radiation beginning on October 2, 2006. Thirty-four total visits, four days per week. This was the beginning of my radiation therapy.

A couple of things landed well in my favor. First of all, I was able to obtain the last treatment time of the day—4:30 p.m. That would mean that I could get a full day of work every day at my office. The hospital was so close to my office that I was able to leave my office at 4:00 p.m. every day and get to the hospital in time for me to change and be on time for my treatment.

The other thing that worked in my favor was that Dr. Strodel indicated that he would be able to use the two tattoos that I had obtained at the large hospital in Chicago. I found out how they were used on day one of my treatments.

Radiation was similar to the CT scans that I had gone through in the past. You are placed on a table that is divided into four sections. There are two small lines of light that emit from the sides of the room. The lines are lined up with the tattoos that you have on your sides. The table you are on is hydraulically raised or lowered to make sure that the tattoos line up exactly with the lines of light. In this fashion, the doctors are making sure that the radiation is targeted exactly where they want it to go. Once the lights are lined up with the tattoos, you are slid into the tube, and the radiation begins. There is a slight humming sound coming from the machine.

Where exactly are they targeting? My prostate was removed back in August of 2003. It seems that they targeted the area where the prostate used to be. They did not know exactly where the reawaken cancer cells were located, but they suspected they were sitting in the area where the prostate used to be.

The first day I had to arrive early so the nurse and doctor could talk to me about clothing and diet. I was assigned a locker to hold my clothes during the time I was in the radiation tube. I walked from the locker area to the radiation room with a towel around my waist. You are naked when you are in the tube.

Dr. Strodel took the time to talk to me about how this was going to impact me. He described it as having a cold, and every day, instead of getting a little better, I would be getting a little worse. He said everyone was different, but he stated that most radiation patients experience mild upset stomachs and a general feeling of being tired all the time. He recommended that I limit the number of salads that I ate so that my stomach and digestive system would be somewhat regular.

The radiation treatments began. As I stated earlier, I was the last patient of the day. I was in the radiation tube for about thirty minutes per day. I fell asleep every single day. It was a nice way to catch a nap. After the daily radiation treatment was completed, the nurse would gently wake me up, and I would walk back to the locker room to change. Once fully dressed, I left the building, but every day, since I was the last patient, the nurses would watch me leave the building and say goodbye. Then they would run to the employee/nurse exit, and we would pretty much leave the building at the same time. It was funny; I would wave to them as they ran to their cars in the employee parking lot about twenty yards away from the patient parking lot.

Radiation was four days per week, Monday to Thursday. I felt pretty good for the first three weeks of the radiation. It had little impact on me, if any, that I could determine. I thought I was going to breeze through this.

Chapter 16

Effects of Radiation

All of a sudden, after the third week, I experienced severe stomach cramps. I had ignored the doctor's recommendation to limit my salad intake. Every day I had my typical lunch—chicken noodle soup, Caesar salad, and iced tea. That was a mistake. Wow, was it a mistake. It was my mistake. On the first day of week four, I went to the bathroom seventeen times. I was wasted! I was weak, and I was pissed. I called the doctor, and he reiterated his previous advice to limit salad consumption. Now he recommended that I go on the BRAT diet—bananas, rice, applesauce, and toast. These are the foods that would calm and not further aggravate my digestive tract.

The last three weeks of my radiation treatment, I ate little other food besides these bland foods. My stomach settled down, and I continued with the radiation treatments. There was a gentleman that I met in the locker room during the treatments. We would chat while we were changing. He was getting dressed in his clothes after his treatment, and I was changing out of my clothes, getting ready for the radiation treatment. We both experienced some discomfort during the radiation. He did not have an upset stomach, but he experienced terrible pains while urinating. I guess I was lucky. I had no pain while urinating.

As I stated earlier, the radiation treatments began on October 2, 2006. The seven-week time frame would end on Friday, November 17, 2006. Oh boy, I was going to be done by Thanksgiving, which was Thursday, November 23, 2006. I was really looking forward to eating the delicious food that my wife, Cory, would cook on that day. Well, I ate the thanksgiving meal and was right back with the same upset stomach that I had during the radiation treatments. It appears that my stomach just was not ready for real heavy food. My stomach calmed down in a few weeks, and I was soon back to my regular eating habits of my past with great satisfaction and glee.

Part 7

(Late 2006 Through Present)

Chapter 17

Life After Radiation

I began a series of meetings with different doctors in six-month intervals. Both Doctor Smith and Doctor Strodel agreed that while they both wanted to see me every six months, I could go to one doctor and then see the other six months later. They would trade information, and in this fashion, both doctors were satisfied.

The first meeting was with Dr. Strodel on December 14, 2006. The result of this meeting consisted of a visual inspection, a digital inspection, and a PSA test. The result of the December 2006 PSA was that the PSA was 0.2. This was excellent news, according to Dr. Strodel. My PSA score in March, June, and July of 2006 was 0.3. It actually could have been higher by the time I started radiation treatments in October. I did not have any PSA tests after July. Dr. Strodel indicated that he was looking for a trend. He said that he would not have been surprised if the PSA stayed the same (0.3) or if there was not any decrease. It was good news as long as it did not go higher. The fact that my PSA score actually went down was excellent.

My next PSA test was administered by Dr. Smith on January 22, 2007. It resulted in a PSA that was decreasing nicely. The value was 0.1.

My PSA score on June 6, 2007, with Dr. Strodel, was 0.1. My PSA score on December 6, 2007, with Dr. Smith, was 0.0. It continued that way for several years. The resultant scores were 0.0 every six months. Finally, in June of 2012, both doctors agreed that there was no need for me to have tests every six months. Dr. Strodel said, "You have graduated. You are welcome to come back if you need us or if you have a question, but there is no need to come back any longer."

I went back to annual checkups with Dr. Smith until he retired in the 2016 to 2018 time frame. During that time, all of my PSA scores have been 0.0. I am truly blessed.

Okay, now everything was working fine. I did not have cancer; my prostate had been removed. I am administering shots to my penis to achieve an erection. My sex life is back to normal, somewhat. I had to change the mix of the tri-mix injection a few times but nothing that caused any real issues. I was hoping to close the book on that part of my life.

Chapter 18

Hematuria Events

I retired in 2013 after thirty-nine years of service working for the utility company in Chicago. One morning in January of 2014, I woke up, and when I went to the toilet to urinate, out came a mixture of thick red pus-type chunks. I was able to urinate, but it was plenty painful. I thought, *Now what!*

This is called *gross hematuria*, and it is the condition where there is blood or red blood cells in the urine. This was more than red blood cells in my case. I had what felt like large chunks of blood coming out of my penis when I tried to urinate.

I immediately went to a branch of the local medical group located in the next town near my house. The doctor performed a cystoscopy, which is a test that allows the doctor to look at the inside of the bladder and the urethra, using a cystoscope, which is a thin camera. It allows the doctor to see areas that do not show up well on x-rays.

It is not very painful, but I felt a burning sensation and felt an urge to urinate when the instrument was inserted and removed.

The doctor also did a CT of my abdomen and my pelvis, with and without contrast. The results were that everything seemed normal.

It happened again in March of 2015. I went through the same process with a cystoscopy. It was found to be without evidence of disease. After these events, it was determined that what I was experiencing was the result of the seven weeks of radiation on my bladder back in 2006. Part of the bladder was damaged during the radiation, and that damaged part finally broke free from the walls of the bladder after eight years. It was pushed out during the normal urination process. It was painful to eliminate, but once it was gone, I was pain-free. The recommendation was that I try to stay hydrated as much as possible so as to minimize a condition in my body that would replicate this activity.

Once again, I was somewhat upset that no one thought to tell me about the potential of this happening. I would have thought that this condition should have been discussed with the patient prior to the seven weeks of radiation to alert him to the potential that this could happen in the future. I was scared out of my mind initially, thinking what was going on! If it would have been discussed with me, I may have been prepared, and then when it did happen, I might have been more understanding of what was going on with my body.

Chapter 19

Summary of Final Results

Since March of 2015, I have been free of any issues in this area of my body. It has been almost eighteen years since I was first diagnosed with prostate cancer. It has been seventeen and a half years since I had my prostate removed. It has been fourteen years since I had seven weeks of radiation. I have been cancer-free for some time now, and I thank all of the doctors and medical personnel who were responsible for giving me this opportunity.

One final suggestion that I have for all men who are going through this is to communicate with their doctor a lot. Ask questions about the success options as well as what happens if something does not go right. Will you be able to have sex again? Will radiation harm you in any way afterward, maybe several years afterward? Had I asked these questions of my doctors, I may have entertained different options. Communication is very important and is a necessity to discover the options and all of the impacts, the various options have on you and your body.

About the Author

William J. Voller, Jr. is one of about 250,000 men who was diagnosed with prostate cancer in 2002. He wrote this book about his experiences with surviving prostate cancer, both with the removal of the prostate in 2003 and with seven weeks of radiation in 2006 when cancer returned. William was born and grew up in the western suburbs of Chicago. He worked in senior management for the local electric utility serving Chicagoland for thirty-nine years. He now lives in Wheaton, Illinois, with his wife. He has two grown children.